Essential Oils Best Collection of Essential Oil Recipes and Blends For Your Body and Soul

Table of content:

Book 2

20+ Recipes For Your Body And Soul
Look Relaxed And Well-Groomed

Essential Oils

Lora Brenner

Essential Oils: 20+ Recipes For Your Body And Soul.

Look Relaxed And Well-Groomed

Introduction

Maybe it looks like there's some really serious scientific stuff going on, but making essential oils actually requires minimal resources and effort but a great amount of patience (not all of us can wait for weeks for the process of infusion to be over).

As you will see from the recipes in the book, you will mostly need only two ingredients – the oil which serves as the so-called carrier oil and the plant whose essential oil you want to extract. When choosing the carrier oil, keep in mind that this should be some light oil with a mild scent.

This is really important because, otherwise, the carrier oil will overpower the fragrance of the plant whose essential oil you want to have. When it comes to the other main ingredient in the recipes, you can use not only flowers but also spices and fruits such as lemons, limes, and oranges. As you can see, there is a wide array of things which you can use to make essential oils.

Now, let's talk about quantities. As you go through the book, you'll notice that there are no set quantities for some recipes. That is because quantities are not that important in extracting essential oils as they may be important in soap making, for instance, where you need to closely follow the quantities recipes call for if you want to get them right.

Here, you can either follow the given quantities or choose the ones you want. In any case, you should remember this – the larger the difference between the quantities of carrier oil and flowers or spices, the less potent the oil will be. Some general rule is to use just enough oil to submerge the other ingredient you are using.

Besides the main ingredients, you'll also need some basic equipment that I'm sure you already have in your kitchen. You will surely need a sieve or cheesecloth for straining the oil, but you should also get dark glass bottles or jars for storing your essential oils. These storage bottles will prevent the light to reach the oil and thus will prolong the shelf-life of essential oils. The oils prepared in this way are usually potent for about 6 months unless specified differently.

I think you are now ready to get on this adventure. Try out these essential oils, check how they would match, and then you can even make your own unique blend.

Chapter 1 – Rose Geranium Oil

Things you'll need:

Geranium flowers, stems, and leaves

Almond, jojoba or light olive oil

How to make the oil?

Step 1: Cut the geranium flowers, stems, and leaves and fill the jar so that it is half or one-third full. Leaves contain the most oil, so you should include lots of these.

Step 2: Use a wooden spoon to gently stir the geranium flowers, leaves, and stems. This serves to release the oils. Make sure that you don't press and crush the contents of the jar.

Step 3: Pour the unscented jojoba oil over the geraniums. You will need as much oil as to cover the geraniums completely.

Step 4: Close the jar and make sure to seal it tightly so as to prevent the air from getting in.

Step 5: Place the jar somewhere outdoors in the sun and leave it there for at least 48 hours. You should give the jar a gentle shake every few hours.

Step 6: Set a funnel over a glass or cup. Place fine cheesecloth over the funnel and pour the oil through it.

Step 7: If you want the oil to be stronger, do not discard the flowers, stems, and leaves but put them back to the strained oil and keep for additional 2 days.

Step 8: When you strain your oil, you should pay attention that there is no any geranium matter in the oil. Otherwise, this matter may decompose and ruin the oil. So, strain the oil several times.

Step 9: Store the oil in a tinted glass bottle. Use a tight-fitting stopper to close the bottle.

Step 10: Place a label on the bottle and write the ingredients as well as the date you made the oil. This is important because the shelf-life of this oil is 6 months.

Chapter 2 – Lavender Oil

Things you'll need:

2-4 cups fresh lavender flowers

Carrier oil (any oil that has a pale color and mild scent. This is important because this oil should not overpower the lavender.)

How to make the oil?

Step 1: Cut the lavender into 1-inch long pieces.

Step 2: Add the lavender flowers to a glass jar. Pour enough carrier oil to cover the flowers and fill the jar leaving about 2 inches from the top.

Step 3: Seal the jar well to prevent air from getting in and keep it in a warm place for at least 48 hours. During this process of brewing, you should mix the contents occasionally.

Step 4: Place a strainer over a glass bowl and strain the oil. Discard the flowers making sure that no plant material remains in the oil. If you want the oil to be stronger, add the flowers to the jar and repeat the same process 2 or more times.

Step 5: Store the oil in a dark glass bottle, seal it well and keep it in a cool place.

The shelf-life of the oil is a year.

Chapter 3 – Lemon Oil

Things you'll need:

1 cup oil, almond, grape seed, coconut oil

5 lemons, try to find organic

How to make the oil?

Step 1: If you can't find organic lemons, first scrub the peels well to make sure that you remove any impurities.

Step 2: Peel the lemons paying attention that there is as little white pith as possible. The oil comes from the yellow part.

Step 3: Pour enough water in your double boiler to cover the bottom.

Step 4: When it begins to simmer, set to the lowest heat. The temperature needs to be really low. Otherwise, the oil may turn rancid as the peels will be scalded.

Step 5: Set your double boiler, add the lemon peels and pour in the oil to cover the peels completely.

Step 6: Keep on low for three hours. Make sure to check the water level and the temperature of the oil.

Step 7: After three hours, place a piece of fine cheesecloth over a glass bowl and strain the oil squeezing the cheesecloth.

Step 8: Store in a dark glass bottle, place a label and keep in a dark and cool place.

Chapter 4 – Rosemary Oil

Things you'll need:

2 cups oil

1 cup rosemary

How to make the oil?

Step 1: Separate the leaves from their stems. You will need a cup of leaves for this recipe.

Step 2: Add the rosemary leaves in a glass jar and pour in the oil. Safflower and sunflower oil are the best options for this recipe because they have a mild scent.

Step 3: Give the jar a gentle shake to make sure that the leaves are submerged completely.

Step 4: Place the jar in a sunny spot and leave to steep for at least one week.

Step 5: place a few layers of cheesecloth over a glass bowl and pour the oil through it.

Step 6: Strain the oil and discard the leaves.

Step 7: Store in a dark glass bottle, make a label and keep in a dark and cool place.

Chapter 5 – Anise Oil

Things you'll need:

2 ounces anise pods

1 cup neutral-flavored oil

How to make the oil?

Step 1: Preheat a stainless-steel pan over medium heat. Once it is hot enough, add the anise pods.

Step 2: Toast the pods for about 5 minutes or until fragrant. Stir the pods frequently.

Step 3: Use a spice grinder to grind the anise pods. Return the ground pods to the saucepan.

Step 4: Pour in a cup of neutral oil and heat for about 10 minutes over medium heat.

Step 5: Remove the pan and leave to cool.

Step 6: Pour this mixture into a glass container. Keep in the fridge for two weeks. During this period, the oil will infuse, and then you can strain it.

Step 7: To strain the oil, use a sieve lined with a few layers of fine cheesecloth.

Step 8: Store the oil in a sterilized glass jar or bottle. Seal the bottle tightly and keep in the fridge.

Step 9: Make a label and use the oil within a month.

Chapter 6 – Chamomile Oil

Things you'll need:

1/2 cup chamomile flowers, completely dried and cleaned from any dirt

¼ cup virgin olive oil

1/4 tablespoon rosemary oil extract

1 tablespoon vitamin E

How to make the oil?

Step 1: First, sterilize a small glass bottle. To do this, prepare boiling water and soak the bottle. Leave it for a few minutes and then leave to dry.

Step 2: Pour in enough olive oil until the bottle is ¾ full.

Step 3: Add the flowers and stir gently so as to soak them completely in the oil. Seal the bottle tightly.

Step 4: Place the bottle in a spot where it will receive direct sunlight for at least 6 hours a day. You should gently take off the lid every day and remove any moisture with a paper towel. Seal the bottle again and shake it well. Repeat this procedure for two weeks.

Step 5: Use fine cheesecloth to strain the oil into another sterilized glass bottle. Discard the flowers.

Step 6: Add the vitamin E and rosemary oil extract and mix well.

Step 7: Make a label and store the oil in a cool and dark place.

Chapter 7 – Cardamom Oil

Things you'll need:

1/2 cup cardamom seeds

Distilled water

How to make the oil?

Step 1: Grind the cardamom seeds until you get fine dust.

Step 2: Place the cardamom powder on a piece of cheesecloth and tie it into a small sachet.

Step 3: Fill your saucepan with distilled water and heat it over medium-high heat.

Step 4: Add the cardamom sachet to the saucepan and leave to simmer for at least 24 hours. The water should be reduced by half.

Step 5: Cover the saucepan with a few layers of cheesecloth and place it in dry daylight. This will help the water get evaporated.

Step 6: Pour this liquid into a glass jar and seal it tightly.

Step 7: Make a label and your cardamom oil is ready.

Chapter 8 – Catnip Oil

Things you'll need:

1 cup olive oil

4 ounces dried catnip

How to make the oil?

Step 1: First, dry the catnip. To do this, secure several cuttings with twine and hang them upside down.

Step 2: Add the dried catnip to a sterilized jar and pour in the olive oil. Secure the lid.

Step 3: Place the jar in a sunny place and leave for a few weeks. Occasionally, give the jar a gentle stir.

Step 4: Place a few layers of cheesecloth over a glass bowl and pour the oil. Strain and discard the catnip. If you want the oil to be stronger, return the flowers to the oil and wait for a few more weeks.

Step 5: Store the oil in a glass bottle, make a label and keep in a cool and dark place.

Chapter 9 – Cinnamon Oil

Things you'll need:

1/2 cup ground cinnamon

2/3 cup olive oil

How to make the oil?

Step 1: Heat a saucepan over medium-high heat.

Step 2: Pour the olive oil, add the cinnamon and stir well.

Step 3: Bring the mixture to the boil and leave to cook for a few minutes.

Step 4: Prepare a strainer lined with a piece of fine cheesecloth, and pour the oil cinnamon mixture through the cheesecloth into a glass bottle.

Step 5: Push down the remaining cinnamon with the spatula to allow the juices to come out. Squeeze the cheesecloth with your hands.

Step 6: Seal the bottle, make a label and store in a cool and dark place.

Chapter 10 – Clove Oil

Things you'll need:

Fresh whole cloves

1/2 cup olive oil

How to make the oil?

Step 1: Grind the cloves in a coffee grinder or mortar. You can tell cloves are fresh by their strong and sharp fresh smell. Use whole cloves instead of buying ground ones because ground cloves deteriorate quickly.

Step 2: Cut a circle in a center of a large coffee filter. The filter should be about 3 inches wide.

Step 3: Cut a piece of cotton string. It should be long enough to tie a knot.

Step 4: Scoop the cloves in the center of the coffee filter. Pinch the sides to make a little sachet and tie the ends with a piece of string.

Step 5: Pour the olive oil into a small jar.

Step 6: Add the sachet with ground cloves to the oil. Shake the jar lightly to make sure that the sachet is completely submerged.

Step 7: Tear a small piece of aluminum foil to form a lid on top of the jar. Also, push the foil a bit inside the jar. This will prevent the oil or steam to escape when you heat it.

Step 8: Heat water in a double boiler.

Step 9: Place the jar into the top section of the double boiler. Let the jar sit and heat in the double boiler for about 45 minutes. The steam will allow the cloves to release their properties into the oil.

Step 10: Take the jar out of the double boiler and place it in a safe place.

Step 11: Allow the bag with the cloves to sit in the oil for one week. The longer you leave them to sit, the stronger the oil will be.

Step 12: Store the oil in a cool and dark place.

Chapter 11 – Eucalyptus Oil

Things you'll need:

2 ounces eucalyptus leaves

Olive oil, for every ¼ ounces of eucalyptus leaves, you will need 1 cup of oil.

How to make the oil?

Step 1: Crush fresh eucalyptus leaves and place them in a crock pot.

Step 2: Add the olive oil.

Step 3: Place the lid on and set the crock pot on low. Allow the mixture to steep for 6 hours.

Step 4: Use a sieve lined with cheesecloth to strain the oil in a dark glass jar.

Step 5: Make a label and seal and store in a cool and dark place.

Step 6: Use within 6 months.

Chapter 12 – Rose Oil

Things you'll need:

4 cups water

1 cup olive oil or jojoba oil

8 cups rose petals

How to make the oil?

Step 1: Pour the water in a saucepan, and when it begins to boil, remove it from the heat.

Step 2: Pour the oil in a glass jar and place the jar in the pan with the warm water.

Step 3: Place the rose petals in a glass bowl and crush them.

Step 4: Add the crushed petals to the jar with the oil. Leave the jar in the warm water.

Step 5: When the water cools, move the jar to a sunny and warm place.

Step 6: Leave to steep for 24 hours.

Step 7: Use a sieve or fine cheesecloth to strain the oil. Discard the rose petals and store the oil in a dark bottle or jar.

Step 8: Add a new batch of crushed rose petals and go through the same process for at least a week.

Step 9: Store the finished product in a dark bottle or jar and keep in a dark and cool place.

Chapter 13 – Sage Oil

Things you'll need:

1 cup fresh sage plant

1/2 cup olive oil

How to make the oil?

Step 1: Place the sage into a freezer bag. Make sure to squeeze out the air, seal the bag and use a rubber mallet to pound the bag to crush the sage.

Step 2: Transfer the crushed sage into a jar and fill it with the olive oil. Put the lid on and place the jar in a warm spot.

Step 3: Leave the jar undisturbed for 48 hours.

Step 4: Strain the oil using a sieve or a piece of fine cheesecloth. Discard the sage leaves and store the oil in a dark glass bottle. If you want to create more potent sage oil, just add a new batch of crushed sage leaves and repeat the process.

Step 5: Make a label and keep the oil in a dark and cool place.

The shelf-life of this sage oil is a year.

Chapter 14 – Jasmine Oil

Things you will need:

Jasmine flowers, dried

Light olive oil*

Use the same amount of the ingredients

How to make the oil?

Step 1: To dry jasmine, you will need to pick the flowers, lay them on a white sheet in full sunlight or and leave them until dried.

Step 2: Fill the jar with the dried flowers.

Step 3: Pour the same amount of oil in the jar so that the flowers are well covered with the oil.

Step 4: Place the lid on and put the jar in a sunny place for about three weeks.

Step 5: Pour the oil through a sieve into a glass bowl.

Step 6: Transfer the oil to a dark jar.

Step 7: Put the lid on and make a label with the date. Store in a cool place.

Chapter 15 – Grapefruit Oil

Things you'll need:

Grapefruits

Carrier oil*

Choose the quantities on your own depending on how much oil you want to make

How to make the oil?

Step 1: To choose the grapefruits for making your essential oil, select those that have a moderately thick rind. Wash the grapefruits thoroughly using warm water and mild detergent. Then, rinse the grapefruits in vinegar.

Step 2: With a zester, remove the rind paying attention not to include the white pith.

Step 3: Layer the rind on a tray and place in a dry and warm place. It will take a few days until the rind dries.

Step 4: Add the dried rind in a crock pot and pour in the carrier oil so that the rind is just submerged. Cover the crock pot, set it on low and leave for at least 8 hours. Another way is to add the grapefruit rind to a Mason jar, seal it and then keep it in a warm and sunny place for at least two weeks.

Step 5: Place a few layers of cheesecloth over a glass bowl.

Step 6: Pour the oil through the cheesecloth and strain squeezing the cheesecloth to get out every drop.

Step 7: Store the oil in a dark glass bottle, seal it well and keep in a cool place.

The shelf-life of grapefruit oil is 3 months.

Chapter 16 – Pine Oil

Things you'll need:

1/ 2 cup sweet almond oil

2 to 3 cups pine tree needles

How to make the oil?

Step 1: Collect fresh pine leaves. Make sure that you use only fresh pine needles from trees. If you use those that have fallen off, you should know that these may spoil your essential oil, as they may cause molds.

Step 2: To prepare the pine needles, wash them thoroughly with warm water. You can even use mild detergent soap. This will remove any impurities. Finally, rinse the needles well.

Step 3: Use clean paper towels to dry the needles.

Step 4: Place the needles in your mortar and pestle and bruise them gently.

Step 5: Add the almond oil to a jar and submerge the needles. Give the jar a good shake.

Step 6: Keep the jar in a warm room for a week. Do not expose the mixture to direct sunlight. You should shake the jar once per day.

Step 7: The next step is to move the jar to a dark place and leave for at least two weeks to ferment. It is important to leave the jar undisturbed during this period.

Step 8: Use a piece of cheesecloth to strain the oil.

Step 9: Store in a dark bottle, seal tightly, make a label and keep in a cool place.

The shelf-life of pine essential oil is about 10 months to a year.

Chapter 17 – Peppermint Oil

Things you'll need:

Fresh peppermint leaves

Olive oil*

Choose the quantities based on what amount of oil you need

How to make the oil?

Step 1: Begin by preparing the peppermint leaves. Wash them thoroughly, and chop or crush them.

Step 2: Add the peppermint leaves in a jar and fill it with the olive oil. It is important that the leaves are completely submerged.

Step 3: Seal the jar and keep it in a sunny spot for 24 hours.

Step 4: Strain the oil through fine cheesecloth and submerge a new batch of crushed peppermint leaves.

Step 5: Seal the jar again and leave in a sunny post for another 24 hours.

Step 6: Repeat these steps for 5 days.

Step 7: After this period, strain the oil into another glass container. Discard the leaves and store the oil in a dark glass bottle.

Step 8: Keep in a dark and cool place.

Chapter 18 – Orange Oil

Things you'll need:

Orange peels

Grain alcohol or vodka

How to make the oil?

Step 1: Scatter the orange peels on your cookie sheet and place somewhere to air dry. It may take you a week to get your peels dry and hard.

Step 2: To chop the dried orange peels, you can use a chopper or food processor. Make sure that you don't over process the peels because they will lose their oil and turn mushy. You just have to chop them into small bits.

Step 3: Transfer the chopped orange peels to a jar and pour in the vodka or grain alcohol.

Step 4: Seal the jar with a tight-fitting lid and leave to sit in a sunny spot for several days. You should also shake the jar a few times a day. You can leave the mixture for even longer, which will lead to extracting more oil.

Step 5: Strain the mixture into another jar using a coffee filter.

Step 6: Place another clean coffee filter on top of this jar and leave for about a week or until the alcohol evaporates. You can strain this oil again if you wish.

Step 7: Store in a dark glass bottle or jar and keep in a cool and dark place.

Chapter 19 – Nutmeg Oil

Things you'll need:

1/2 cup grapeseed oil

3/4 cup whole nutmegs

How to make the oil?

Step 1: Add the nutmeg to the mortar and pestle and crush the nutmegs until they release their fragrance.

Step 2: You should have ½ cup of these crushed nutmegs. Add them to a jar.

Step 3: Pour the oil over the nutmegs in the jar so that they are submerged.

Step 4: Seal the jar well and give it a good shake.

Step 5: Place the jar in a place with direct sunlight and leave it there for at least 48 hours. You should shake the jar every 12 hours.

Step 6: Use a strainer or cheesecloth to strain the oil in a jar or glass bowl. Discard the crushed nutmeg.

Step 7: Pour the strained oil back to the jar and add another batch of nutmegs.

Step 8: Leave the jar in a warm place again for 48 hours. Strain the oil and if you want the oil to be stronger, repeat these steps again.

Step 9: Store the strained oil in a dark bottle. Seal it well and place in a dark and cool place.

If stored properly, the oil can be used within 6 months to a year.

Chapter 20 – Lime Oil

Things you will need:

2 cups olive oil

4 limes

2 Kaffir lime leaves

How to make the oil?

Step 1: Pour the olive oil in a saucepan and heat over medium heat.

Step 2: To prepare the limes, first wash them thoroughly. With a zester or paring knife, remove the lime zest cutting it into strips. Make sure that you don't cut into the pith.

Step 3: Add the Kaffir leaves and lime zest to the oil in the saucepan. Leave the mixture to simmer over medium heat.

Step 4: After 10 minutes, remove the saucepan and leave it to sit covered and steep for 2 and a half hours.

Step 5: Strain the oil with a fine-mesh sieve into an airtight container.

Step 6: Store the essential oil in a dark and cool place.

Use this oil within two weeks.

Chapter 21 – Vanilla Oil

Things you'll need:

Whole vanilla pods

8 ounces carrier oil (jojoba, apricot, almond)

How to make the oil?

Step 1: First, prepare the vanilla pods. Chop them and remove the seeds.

Step 2: Pour the carrier oil in a glass jar. Add the chopped vanilla pods and stir to submerge them.

Step 3: Leave to sit in a warm place for a week to infuse. If you want your vanilla oil to be stronger, leave it to infuse longer.

Step 4: Use a strainer or fine cheesecloth to strain the oil in a dark glass jar or bottle.

Step 5: Seal the container and store in a cool and dark place.

Note: If you wish, you can leave the pods, but in that case, you should use an airtight container to prevent oxidation. Also, make sure that the pods are completely immersed in the oil.

Chapter 22 – Sandalwood Oil

Things you'll need:

1 cup carrier oil (olive or jojoba)

1/4 ounce sandalwood powder

How to make the oil?

Step 1: Preheat your oven to 200F.

Step 2: Add the oil to a saucepan and mix in the sandalwood powder.

Step 3: Place the lid on the pan and put the saucepan in the preheated oven.

Step 4: Leave the oil and sandalwood mixture to cook for about 2 to 4 hours.

Step 5: To prevent the oil from burning, stir the mixture frequently.

Step 6: Place a few layers of cheesecloth over a jar and pour the mixture through it. Squeeze the cheesecloth to strain the oil.

Step 7: Make a label and store in a cool and dark place.

Use this oil within 6 months.

Chapter 23 – Fennel Oil

Things you'll need:

2 cups olive oil

2 fennel bulbs

How to make the oil?

Step 1: Begin by cleaning the fennel bulbs. Wash them thoroughly under cool water.

Step 2: Since you will use only the bulbs, trim the stems and leaves. Then, chop the bulbs into small cubes.

Step 3: Pour the olive oil in a saucepan and add the fennel cubes.

Step 4: Place the saucepan over high heat and when the mixture begins to boil, reduce the heat and leave to simmer for an hour.

Step 5: Use a sieve to strain the oil. Press the fennel solids with your flexible spatula to squeeze out the oil.

Step 6: Store the oil in a dark bottle, seal and keep in your fridge.

Conclusion

No, your essential oil adventure is not over! Now, you know the basics of how to make essential oils at home in a few easy steps. The recipes covered in the book give you a good foundation to continue exploring various essential oil blends. This process of extracting essential oils requires minimal effort but is really rewarding, as it gives you not only products that you can use in your diffuser to freshen up your home, but they also have numerous health and beauty benefits. After the recipe you can find here, I bet you feel inspired to make your own unique blend of essential oils?

Essential Oils

45

Wonderful

Summer

Diffuser Recipes

Lora Brenner

Essential Oils

45 Wonderful Summer Diffuser Blends

Introduction

It appears that nowadays we have forgotten to stop for a moment and listen to our bodies and what our senses are telling us. Scent appears to be the sense to which we do not pay enough attention. So, we often forget what a strong impact it can have on the body, soul, and mind. One very simple way of reconnecting these three elements is diffusing essential oils.

The term diffusion refers to the tendency of molecules to spread out and occupy an available space. Molecules in liquids typically diffuse from an environment with a high concentration to the one where there is less concentration.

Overheating essential oils may produce a stronger aroma, but this is actually not a good way of diffusing oils. Instead, this actually makes the oils less beneficial. Two great and effective methods of diffusing essential oils are the candle and ultrasonic diffusing. Let's take a look.

Candle & Ultrasonic Diffusers

Candle diffusers are typically metal or ceramic and consist of a bowl or dish for essential oils and an opening where a candle can be inserted. These diffusers can be found in various shapes, from simple ones to those that can have a decorative purpose as well since they look really beautiful as the candle gently flickers away.

Candle diffusers utilize the heat that the candle produces to gently warm the mixture of water and essential.

This vaporizes the essential oil(s) and supports the diffusion process. Candle diffusers are not that pricey and do not require batteries or electricity. However, it is advised not to leave the candle lit overnight or unattended.

Ultrasonic diffusers combine the best of air purifiers, humidifiers, atomizers, and aromatherapy diffusers into one device. They work so as to break an essential oil into millions of particles and then disperse them into the air. The moment these oil droplets leave the diffuser, the mist turns into a vapor that spreads evenly across the room.

They can also be found in various shapes and colors, and some even feature colored lights. Since these diffusers do not use heat but ultrasonic vibrations, they can also add moisture into the air. Ultrasonic diffusers are safer to use because they can work all day and night since there is no naked flame.

Essential Oils

Besides their intoxicating fragrance, essential oils can also improve concentration, uplift mood, relax, and boost energy. Moreover, certain oils can have other benefits as well, such as relieving the symptoms of insomnia, headaches, and asthma. Also, some oils, such as lemon and rosemary essential oils, can improve your immune system and relieve stress. Many essential oils have also proven to relieve depression and anxiety.

There's a whole variety of essential oils that you can use – eucalyptus, basil, rose, geranium, white fir, lemon, thyme, lavender, rosemary, chamomile, lime, spearmint, etc. Moreover, you can experiment and make various oil blends and get a unique fragrance with amazing health benefits. Since essential oils are very concentrated and powerful, you will need just a few drops, and it will go a long way.

Once you get your oil diffuser, you just have to choose essential oils, and you are ready to go.

Chapter 1 – Fresh & Clean

Ingredients:

2 drops Rosemary essential oil

2 drops Lemon essential oil

2 drops Lavender essential oil

Instructions for ultrasonic diffusers:

1. Pour enough lukewarm water to fill the diffuser dish half the fill-line or up to the fill-line depending on how strong you want the fragrance to be.

2. Add the rosemary, lemon, and lavender essential oils and put the lid back on. Press the power button to turn the diffuser on.

Instructions for candle diffusers:

1. Pour a few tablespoons of lukewarm water into the dish.

2. Add the essential oils and light the candle.

Chapter 2 – Let's Focus

Ingredients:

2 drops Peppermint essential oil

2 drops Wild Orange essential oil

Instructions for ultrasonic diffusers:

1. Pour enough lukewarm water to fill the diffuser dish half the fill-line or up to the fill-line depending on how strong you want the fragrance to be.

2. Add the peppermint and wild orange essential oils and put the lid back on. Press the power button to turn the diffuser on.

Instructions for candle diffusers:

1. Pour a few tablespoons of lukewarm water into the dish.

2. Add the peppermint and wild orange essential oils and light the candle.

Chapter 3 – Eliminate Those Odors

Ingredients:

1 drop Lime essential oil

1 drop Tea Tree essential oil

2 drops Lemon essential oil

1 drop Cilantro essential oil

Instructions for ultrasonic diffusers:

1. Pour enough lukewarm water to fill the diffuser dish half the fill-line or up to the fill-line depending on how strong you want the fragrance to be.

2. Add the lime, tea tree, lemon, and cilantro essential oils and put the lid back on. Press the power button to turn the diffuser on.

Instructions for candle diffusers:

1. Pour a few tablespoons of lukewarm water into the dish.

2. Add the lime, tea tree, lemon, and cilantro essential oils and light the candle.

Chapter 4 – Citrus Explosion

Ingredients:

1 drop Grapefruit essential oil

2 drops Wild Orange essential oil

1 drop Lemon essential oil

1 drop Lime essential oil

Instructions for ultrasonic diffusers:

1. Pour enough lukewarm water to fill the diffuser dish half the fill-line or up to the fill-line depending on how strong you want the fragrance to be.

2. Add the grapefruit, wild orange, lemon, and lime essential oils and put the lid back on. Press the power button to turn the diffuser on.

Instructions for candle diffusers:

1. Pour a few tablespoons of lukewarm water into the dish.

2. Add the grapefruit, wild orange, lemon, and lime essential oils and light the candle.

Chapter 5 – Take A Deep Breath

Ingredients:

1 drop Patchouli essential oil

1 drop Bergamot essential oil

1 drop Ylang Ylang essential oil

Instructions for ultrasonic diffusers:

1. Pour enough lukewarm water to fill the diffuser dish half the fill-line or up to the fill-line depending on how strong you want the fragrance to be.

2. Add the patchouli, bergamot, and ylang ylang essential oils and put the lid back on. Press the power button to turn the diffuser on.

Instructions for candle diffusers:

1. Pour a few tablespoons of lukewarm water into the dish.

2. Add the patchouli, bergamot, and ylang ylang essential oils and light the candle.

Chapter 6 – Flower Garden

Ingredients:

2 drops Lavender essential oil

1 drop Geranium essential oil

2 drops Roman Chamomile essential oil

Instructions for ultrasonic diffusers:

1. Pour enough lukewarm water to fill the diffuser dish half the fill-line or up to the fill-line depending on how strong you want the fragrance to be.

2. Add the lavender, geranium, and roman chamomile essential oils and put the lid back on. Press the power button to turn the diffuser on.

Instructions for candle diffusers:

1. Pour a few tablespoons of lukewarm water into the dish.

2. Add the lavender, geranium, and roman chamomile essential oils and light the candle.

Chapter 7 – Man-Cave Blend

Ingredients:

2 drops Cypress essential oil

2 drops White Fir essential oil

2 drops Wintergreen essential oil

Instructions for ultrasonic diffusers:

1. Pour enough lukewarm water to fill the diffuser dish half the fill-line or up to the fill-line depending on how strong you want the fragrance to be.

2. Add the cypress, white fir, and wintergreen essential oils and put the lid back on. Press the power button to turn the diffuser on.

Instructions for candle diffusers:

1. Pour a few tablespoons of lukewarm water into the dish.

2. Add the cypress, white fir, and wintergreen essential oils and light the candle.

Chapter 8 – Bug Repellent Blend

Ingredients:

1 drop Eucalyptus essential oil

1 drop Thyme essential oil

1 drop Lemongrass essential oil

1 drop Basil essential oil

Instructions for ultrasonic diffusers:

1. Pour enough lukewarm water to fill the diffuser dish half the fill-line or up to the fill-line depending on how strong you want the fragrance to be.

2. Add the eucalyptus, thyme, lemongrass, and basil essential oils and put the lid back on. Press the power button to turn the diffuser on.

Instructions for candle diffusers:

1. Pour a few tablespoons of lukewarm water into the dish.

2. Add the eucalyptus, thyme, lemongrass, and basil essential oils and light the candle.

Chapter 9 – Spicy Citrus

Ingredients:

2 drops Cinnamon Bark essential oil

3 drops Wild Orange essential oil

1 drop Clove essential oil

Instructions for ultrasonic diffusers:

1. Pour enough lukewarm water to fill the diffuser dish half the fill-line or up to the fill-line depending on how strong you want the fragrance to be.

2. Add the cinnamon, wild orange, and clove essential oils and put the lid back on. Press the power button to turn the diffuser on.

Instructions for candle diffusers:

1. Pour a few tablespoons of lukewarm water into the dish.

2. Add the cinnamon, wild orange, and clove essential oils and light the candle.

Chapter 10 – Bye-Bye Stress

Ingredients:

2 drops Bergamot essential oil

2 drops Frankincense essential oil

Instructions for ultrasonic diffusers:

1. Pour enough lukewarm water to fill the diffuser dish half the fill-line or up to the fill-line depending on how strong you want the fragrance to be.

2. Add the cinnamon, wild orange, and clove essential oils and put the lid back on. Press the power button to turn the diffuser on.

Instructions for candle diffusers:

1. Pour a few tablespoons of lukewarm water into the dish.

2. Add the cinnamon, wild orange, and clove essential oils and light the candle.

Chapter 11 – Count To Ten & Relax

Ingredients:

2 drops Bergamot essential oil

1 drop Roman Chamomile essential oil

2 drops Orange essential oil

Instructions for ultrasonic diffusers:

1. Pour enough lukewarm water to fill the diffuser dish half the fill-line or up to the fill-line depending on how strong you want the fragrance to be.

2. Add the bergamot, roman chamomile, and orange essential oils and put the lid back on. Press the power button to turn the diffuser on.

Instructions for candle diffusers:

1. Pour a few tablespoons of lukewarm water into the dish.

2. Add the bergamot, roman chamomile, and orange essential oils and light the candle.

Chapter 12 – Anxiety Relief

Ingredients:

2 drops Mandarin essential oil

1 drop Lavender essential oil

1 drop Rose essential oil

1 drop Vetiver essential oil

Instructions for ultrasonic diffusers:

1. Pour enough lukewarm water to fill the diffuser dish half the fill-line or up to the fill-line depending on how strong you want the fragrance to be.

2. Add the mandarin, lavender, rose, and vetiver essential oils and put the lid back on. Press the power button to turn the diffuser on.

Instructions for candle diffusers:

1. Pour a few tablespoons of lukewarm water into the dish.

2. Add the mandarin, lavender, rose, and vetiver essential oils and light the candle.

Chapter 13 – Flu-Symptom Relief

Ingredients:

3 drops Ravintsara essential oil

5 drops Siberian Fir essential oil

4 drops Lemon essential oil

Instructions for ultrasonic diffusers:

1. Pour enough lukewarm water to fill the diffuser dish half the fill-line or up to the fill-line depending on how strong you want the fragrance to be.

2. Add the ravintsara, Siberian fir, and lemon essential oils and put the lid back on. Press the power button to turn the diffuser on.

Instructions for candle diffusers:

1. Pour a few tablespoons of lukewarm water into the dish.

2. Add the ravintsara, Siberian fir, and lemon essential oils and light the candle.

Chapter 14 – Summer Sunshine

Ingredients:

2 drops Lemon essential oil

3 drops Grapefruit essential oil

3 drops Orange essential oil

1 drop Bergamot essential oil

Instructions for ultrasonic diffusers:

1. Pour enough lukewarm water to fill the diffuser dish half the fill-line or up to the fill-line depending on how strong you want the fragrance to be.

2. Add the lemon, grapefruit, orange, and bergamot essential oils and put the lid back on. Press the power button to turn the diffuser on.

Instructions for candle diffusers:

1. Pour a few tablespoons of lukewarm water into the dish.

2. Add the lemon, grapefruit, orange, and bergamot essential oils and light the candle.

Chapter 15 – Must Concentrate

Ingredients:

3 drops Lemon essential oil

3 drops Rosemary essential oil

1 drops Peppermint essential oil

Instructions for ultrasonic diffusers:

1. Pour enough lukewarm water to fill the diffuser dish half the fill-line or up to the fill-line depending on how strong you want the fragrance to be.

2. Add the lemon, rosemary, and peppermint essential oils and put the lid back on. Press the power button to turn the diffuser on.

Instructions for candle diffusers:

1. Pour a few tablespoons of lukewarm water into the dish.

2. Add the lemon, rosemary, and peppermint essential oils and light the candle.

Chapter 16 – Sinus Headache Relief

Ingredients:

2 drops Eucalyptus Blue essential oil

4 drops Geranium essential oil

5 drops Tea Tree essential oil

9 drops Rosemary essential oil

3 drops Peppermint essential oil

2 drops Lavender essential oil

Instructions for ultrasonic diffusers:

1. Pour enough lukewarm water to fill the diffuser dish half the fill-line or up to the fill-line depending on how strong you want the fragrance to be.

2. Add the eucalyptus blue, geranium, tea tree, rosemary, peppermint, and lavender essential oils and put the lid back on. Press the power button to turn the diffuser on.

Instructions for candle diffusers:

1. Pour a few tablespoons of lukewarm water into the dish.

2. Add the eucalyptus blue, geranium, tea tree, rosemary, peppermint, and lavender essential oils and light the candle.

Chapter 17 – Go On Vacation

Ingredients:

2 drops Orange essential oil

3 drops Stressaway essential oil

1 drop Sandalwood essential oil

Instructions for ultrasonic diffusers:

1. Pour enough lukewarm water to fill the diffuser dish half the fill-line or up to the fill-line depending on how strong you want the fragrance to be.

2. Add the orange, stressaway, and sandalwood essential oils and put the lid back on. Press the power button to turn the diffuser on.

Instructions for candle diffusers:

1. Pour a few tablespoons of lukewarm water into the dish.

2. Add the orange, stressaway, and sandalwood essential oils and light the candle.

Chapter 18 – Relaxing Spa

Ingredients:

3 drops Citrus Fresh essential oil

3 drops Lavender essential oil

Instructions for ultrasonic diffusers:

1. Pour enough lukewarm water to fill the diffuser dish half the fill-line or up to the fill-line depending on how strong you want the fragrance to be.

2. Add the citrus fresh and lavender essential oils and put the lid back on. Press the power button to turn the diffuser on.

Instructions for candle diffusers:

1. Pour a few tablespoons of lukewarm water into the dish.
2. Add the citrus fresh and lavender essential oils and light the candle.

Chapter 19 – Anger Management

Ingredients:

4 drops Citrus Fresh essential oil

4 drops Release essential oil

4 drops Peace and Calming essential oil

Instructions for ultrasonic diffusers:

1. Pour enough lukewarm water to fill the diffuser dish half the fill-line or up to the fill-line depending on how strong you want the fragrance to be.

2. Add the citrus fresh, release, and peace and calming essential oils and put the lid back on. Press the power button to turn the diffuser on.

Instructions for candle diffusers:

1. Pour a few tablespoons of lukewarm water into the dish.

2. Add the citrus fresh, release, and peace and calming essential oils and light the candle.

Chapter 20 – Citrus Forest

Ingredients:

1 drop Bergamot essential oil

2 drops Lemon essential oil

2 drops Lime essential oil

1 drop Orange essential oil

1 drop White Fir essential oil

Instructions for ultrasonic diffusers:

1. Pour enough lukewarm water to fill the diffuser dish half the fill-line or up to the fill-line depending on how strong you want the fragrance to be.

2. Add the bergamot, lemon, lime, orange, and white fir essential oils and put the lid back on. Press the power button to turn the diffuser on.

Instructions for candle diffusers:

1. Pour a few tablespoons of lukewarm water into the dish.

2. Add the bergamot, lemon, lime, orange, and white fir essential oils and light the candle.

Chapter 21 – Morning Clarity

Ingredients:

2 drops Spearmint essential oil

3 drops Peppermint essential oil

1 drop Wintergreen essential oil

Instructions for ultrasonic diffusers:

1. Pour enough lukewarm water to fill the diffuser dish half the fill-line or up to the fill-line depending on how strong you want the fragrance to be.

2. Add the spearmint, peppermint, and wintergreen essential oils and put the lid back on. Press the power button to turn the diffuser on.

Instructions for candle diffusers:

1. Pour a few tablespoons of lukewarm water into the dish.

2. Add the spearmint, peppermint, and wintergreen essential oils and light the candle.

Chapter 22 – Soothing Blend

Ingredients:

6 drops Grapefruit essential oil

6 drops Lime essential oil

6 drops Bergamot essential oil

2 drops Sandalwood essential oils

4 drops Ginger essential oil

Instructions for ultrasonic diffusers:

1. Pour enough lukewarm water to fill the diffuser dish half the fill-line or up to the fill-line depending on how strong you want the fragrance to be.

2. Add the grapefruit, lime, bergamot, sandalwood, and ginger essential oils and put the lid back on. Press the power button to turn the diffuser on.

Instructions for candle diffusers:

1. Pour a few tablespoons of lukewarm water into the dish.

2. Add the grapefruit, lime, bergamot, sandalwood, and ginger essential oils and light the candle.

Chapter 23 – Remember Winter

Ingredients:

3 drops Wild Orange essential oils

3 drops White Fir essential oils

2 drop Wintergreen essential oils

Instructions for ultrasonic diffusers:

1. Pour enough lukewarm water to fill the diffuser dish half the fill-line or up to the fill-line depending on how strong you want the fragrance to be.

2. Add the wild orange, white fir, and wintergreen essential oils and put the lid back on. Press the power button to turn the diffuser on.

Instructions for candle diffusers:

1. Pour a few tablespoons of lukewarm water into the dish.

2. Add the wild orange, white fir, and wintergreen essential oils and light the candle.

Chapter 24 – Autumn-Infused Air

Ingredients:

3 drops Cinnamon essential oil

4 drops Wild Orange essential oil

3 drops Ginger essential oil

Instructions for ultrasonic diffusers:

1. Pour enough lukewarm water to fill the diffuser dish half the fill-line or up to the fill-line depending on how strong you want the fragrance to be.

2. Add the cinnamon, wild orange, and ginger essential oils and put the lid back on. Press the power button to turn the diffuser on.

Instructions for candle diffusers:

1. Pour a few tablespoons of lukewarm water into the dish.

2. Add the cinnamon, wild orange, and ginger essential oils and light the candle.

Chapter 25 – Common Cold Relief

Ingredients:

3 drops Cypress essential oil

4 drops Eucalyptus essential oil

5 drops Rosemary essential oil

4 drops Peppermint essential oil

2 drops Lemon essential oil

Instructions for ultrasonic diffusers:

1. Pour enough lukewarm water to fill the diffuser dish half the fill-line or up to the fill-line depending on how strong you want the fragrance to be.

2. Add the cypress, eucalyptus, rosemary, peppermint, and lemon essential oils and put the lid back on. Press the power button to turn the diffuser on.

Instructions for candle diffusers:

1. Pour a few tablespoons of lukewarm water into the dish.

2. Add the cypress, eucalyptus, rosemary, peppermint, and lemon essential oils and light the candle.

Chapter 26 – Fresh Air

Ingredients:

3 drops Lemon essential oil

3 drops Tea Tree essential oil

3 drops Lime essential oil

Instructions for ultrasonic diffusers:

1. Pour enough lukewarm water to fill the diffuser dish half the fill-line or up to the fill-line depending on how strong you want the fragrance to be.

2. Add the lemon, tea tree, and lime essential oils and put the lid back on. Press the power button to turn the diffuser on.

Instructions for candle diffusers:

1. Pour a few tablespoons of lukewarm water into the dish.

2. Add the lemon, tea tree, and lime essential oils and light the candle.

Chapter 27 – Headache Relief

Ingredients:

4 drops Eucalyptus essential oil

6 drops Peppermint essential oil

2 drops Myrrh essential oil

Instructions for ultrasonic diffusers:

1. Pour enough lukewarm water to fill the diffuser dish half the fill-line or up to the fill-line depending on how strong you want the fragrance to be.

2. Add the eucalyptus, peppermint, and myrrh essential oils and put the lid back on. Press the power button to turn the diffuser on.

Instructions for candle diffusers:

1. Pour a few tablespoons of lukewarm water into the dish.

2. Add the eucalyptus, peppermint, and myrrh essential oils and light the candle.

Chapter 28 – It's Time To Sleep

Ingredients:

1 drop Orange essential oil

2 drops Marjoram essential oil

3 drops Lavender essential oil

1 drop Roman Chamomile essential oil

Instructions for ultrasonic diffusers:

1. Pour enough lukewarm water to fill the diffuser dish half the fill-line or up to the fill-line depending on how strong you want the fragrance to be.

2. Add the orange, marjoram, lavender, and roman chamomile essential oils and put the lid back on. Press the power button to turn the diffuser on.

Instructions for candle diffusers:

1. Pour a few tablespoons of lukewarm water into the dish.

2. Add the orange, marjoram, lavender, and roman chamomile essential oils and light the candle.

Chapter 29 – Stay Healthy

Ingredients:

2 drop Cinnamon essential oil

2 drop Clove essential oil

2 drop Rosemary essential oil

2 drop Eucalyptus essential oil

2 drop Wild Orange essential oil

Instructions for ultrasonic diffusers:

1. Pour enough lukewarm water to fill the diffuser dish half the fill-line or up to the fill-line depending on how strong you want the fragrance to be.

2. Add the cinnamon, clove, rosemary, eucalyptus, and wild orange essential oils and put the lid back on. Press the power button to turn the diffuser on.

Instructions for candle diffusers:

1. Pour a few tablespoons of lukewarm water into the dish.

2. Add the cinnamon, clove, rosemary, eucalyptus, and wild orange essential oils and light the candle.

Chapter 30 – Immune Booster

Ingredients:

2 drops Eucalyptus essential oil

2 drops Peppermint essential oil

1 drop Lime essential oil

2 drops Lemon essential oil

1 drop Rosemary essential oil

1 drop Clove essential oil

Instructions for ultrasonic diffusers:

1. Pour enough lukewarm water to fill the diffuser dish half the fill-line or up to the fill-line depending on how strong you want the fragrance to be.

2. Add the eucalyptus, peppermint, lime, lemon, rosemary, and clove essential oils and put the lid back on. Press the power button to turn the diffuser on.

Instructions for candle diffusers:

1. Pour a few tablespoons of lukewarm water into the dish.

2. Add the eucalyptus, peppermint, lime, lemon, rosemary, and clove essential oils and light the candle.

Chapter 31 – Relax

Ingredients:

3 drops Frankincense essential oil

3 drops Bergamot essential oil

3 drops Elevation essential oil

Instructions for ultrasonic diffusers:

1. Pour enough lukewarm water to fill the diffuser dish half the fill-line or up to the fill-line depending on how strong you want the fragrance to be.

2. Add the frankincense, bergamot, and elevation essential oils and put the lid back on. Press the power button to turn the diffuser on.

Instructions for candle diffusers:

1. Pour a few tablespoons of lukewarm water into the dish.

2. Add the frankincense, bergamot, and elevation essential oils and light the candle.

Chapter 32 – Take It Easy

Ingredients:

1 drop Clary Sage essential oil

2 drops Vetiver essential oil

4 drops Lavender essential oil

1 drop Lemon essential oil

Instructions for ultrasonic diffusers:

1. Pour enough lukewarm water to fill the diffuser dish half the fill-line or up to the fill-line depending on how strong you want the fragrance to be.

2. Add the clary sage, vetiver, lavender, and lemon essential oils and put the lid back on. Press the power button to turn the diffuser on.

Instructions for candle diffusers:

1. Pour a few tablespoons of lukewarm water into the dish.

2. Add the clary sage, vetiver, lavender, and lemon essential oils and light the candle.

Chapter 33 – Night Blossom

Ingredients:

3 drops Jasmine essential oil

1 drop Lemon Myrtle essential oil

1 drop Patchouli essential oil

Instructions for ultrasonic diffusers:

1. Pour enough lukewarm water to fill the diffuser dish half the fill-line or up to the fill-line depending on how strong you want the fragrance to be.

2. Add the jasmine, lemon myrtle, and patchouli essential oils and put the lid back on. Press the power button to turn the diffuser on.

Instructions for candle diffusers:

1. Pour a few tablespoons of lukewarm water into the dish.

2. Add the jasmine, lemon myrtle, and patchouli essential oils and light the candle.

Chapter 34 – Be Happy

Ingredients:

2 drops Wild Orange essential oil

2 drops Peppermint essential oil

2 drops Frankincense essential oil

2 drops Lime essential oil

Instructions for ultrasonic diffusers:

1. Pour enough lukewarm water to fill the diffuser dish half the fill-line or up to the fill-line depending on how strong you want the fragrance to be.

2. Add the wild orange, peppermint, frankincense, and lime essential oils and put the lid back on. Press the power button to turn the diffuser on.

Instructions for candle diffusers:

1. Pour a few tablespoons of lukewarm water into the dish.

2. Add the wild orange, peppermint, frankincense, and lime essential oils and light the candle.

Chapter 35 – Calm Down

Ingredients:

2 drops Clary Sage essential oil

3 drops Geranium essential oil

3 drops Lavender essential oil

2 drops Roman Chamomile essential oil

2 drops Ylang Ylang essential oil

Instructions for ultrasonic diffusers:

1. Pour enough lukewarm water to fill the diffuser dish half the fill-line or up to the fill-line depending on how strong you want the fragrance to be.

2. Add the clary sage, geranium, lavender, roman chamomile, and ylang ylang essential oils and put the lid back on. Press the power button to turn the diffuser on.

Instructions for candle diffusers:

1. Pour a few tablespoons of lukewarm water into the dish.

2. Add the clary sage, geranium, lavender, roman chamomile, and ylang ylang essential oils and light the candle.

Chapter 36 – Stress Away

Ingredients:

2 drops Ylang Ylang essential oil

3 drops Clary Sage essential oil

4 drops Lavender essential oil

1 drop Marjoram essential oil

Instructions for ultrasonic diffusers:

1. Pour enough lukewarm water to fill the diffuser dish half the fill-line or up to the fill-line depending on how strong you want the fragrance to be.

2. Add the ylang ylang, clary sage, lavender, and marjoram essential oils and put the lid back on. Press the power button to turn the diffuser on.

Instructions for candle diffusers:

1. Pour a few tablespoons of lukewarm water into the dish.

2. Add the ylang ylang, clary sage, lavender, and marjoram essential oils and light the candle.

Chapter 37 – Say Goodbye To Headaches

Ingredients:

2 drops Thyme essential oil

2 drops Peppermint essential oil

2 drops Marjoram essential oil

2 drops Rosemary essential oil

2 drops Lavender essential oil

Instructions for ultrasonic diffusers:

1. Pour enough lukewarm water to fill the diffuser dish half the fill-line or up to the fill-line depending on how strong you want the fragrance to be.

2. Add the thyme, peppermint, marjoram, rosemary, and lavender essential oils and put the lid back on. Press the power button to turn the diffuser on.

Instructions for candle diffusers:

1. Pour a few tablespoons of lukewarm water into the dish.

2. Add the thyme, peppermint, marjoram, rosemary, and lavender essential oils and light the candle.

Chapter 38 – Allergy Relief

Ingredients:

3 drops Lavender essential oil

3 drops Peppermint essential oil

3 drops Lemon essential oil

Instructions for ultrasonic diffusers:

1. Pour enough lukewarm water to fill the diffuser dish half the fill-line or up to the fill-line depending on how strong you want the fragrance to be.

2. Add the lavender, peppermint, and lemon essential oils and put the lid back on. Press the power button to turn the diffuser on.

Instructions for candle diffusers:

1. Pour a few tablespoons of lukewarm water into the dish.

2. Add the lavender, peppermint, and lemon essential oils and light the candle.

Chapter 39 – It's Summertime

Ingredients:

2 drops Lemon essential oil

3 drops Lavender essential oil

3 drops Grapefruit essential oil

2 drops Spearmint essential oil

Instructions for ultrasonic diffusers:

1. Pour enough lukewarm water to fill the diffuser dish half the fill-line or up to the fill-line depending on how strong you want the fragrance to be.

2. Add the lemon, lavender, grapefruit, and spearmint essential oils and put the lid back on. Press the power button to turn the diffuser on.

Instructions for candle diffusers:

1. Pour a few tablespoons of lukewarm water into the dish.

2. Add the lemon, lavender, grapefruit, and spearmint essential oils and light the candle.

Chapter 40 – Immune System Booster

Ingredients:

1 drop Cinnamon Bark essential oil

1 drop Clove essential oil

1 drop Rosemary essential oil

1 drop Eucalyptus essential oil

1 drop Wild Orange essential oil

Instructions for ultrasonic diffusers:

1. Pour enough lukewarm water to fill the diffuser dish half the fill-line or up to the fill-line depending on how strong you want the fragrance to be.

2. Add the cinnamon, clove, rosemary, eucalyptus, wild orange essential oils and put the lid back on. Press the power button to turn the diffuser on.

Instructions for candle diffusers:

1. Pour a few tablespoons of lukewarm water into the dish.

2. Add the cinnamon, clove, rosemary, eucalyptus, wild orange essential oils and light the candle.

Chapter 41 – Good Morning

Ingredients:

4 drops Peppermint essential oil

4 drops Wild Orange essential oil

Instructions for ultrasonic diffusers:

1. Pour enough lukewarm water to fill the diffuser dish half the fill-line or up to the fill-line depending on how strong you want the fragrance to be.

2. Add the peppermint and wild orange essential oils and put the lid back on. Press the power button to turn the diffuser on.

Instructions for candle diffusers:

1. Pour a few tablespoons of lukewarm water into the dish.

2. Add the peppermint and wild orange essential oils and light the candle.

Chapter 42 – Boost Your Energy

Ingredients:

2 drops Frankincense essential oil

2 drops Wild Orange essential oil

2 drops Cinnamon essential oil

Instructions for ultrasonic diffusers:

1. Pour enough lukewarm water to fill the diffuser dish half the fill-line or up to the fill-line depending on how strong you want the fragrance to be.

2. Add the frankincense, wild orange, cinnamon essential oils and put the lid back on. Press the power button to turn the diffuser on.

Instructions for candle diffusers:

1. Pour a few tablespoons of lukewarm water into the dish.

2. Add the frankincense, wild orange, cinnamon essential oils and light the candle.

Chapter 43 – Sunset

Ingredients:

2 drops Ylang Ylang essential oil

2 drops Cedarwood essential oil

1 drop Jasmine essential oil

Instructions for ultrasonic diffusers:

1. Pour enough lukewarm water to fill the diffuser dish half the fill-line or up to the fill-line depending on how strong you want the fragrance to be.

2. Add the ylang ylang, cedarwood, and jasmine essential oils and put the lid back on. Press the power button to turn the diffuser on.

Instructions for candle diffusers:

1. Pour a few tablespoons of lukewarm water into the dish.

2. Add the ylang ylang, cedarwood, and jasmine essential oils and light the candle.

Chapter 44 – Candy Store

Ingredients:

2 drop Wintergreen essential oil

2 drops Wild Orange essential oil

Instructions for ultrasonic diffusers:

1. Pour enough lukewarm water to fill the diffuser dish half the fill-line or up to the fill-line depending on how strong you want the fragrance to be.

2. Add the wintergreen and wild orange essential oils and put the lid back on. Press the power button to turn the diffuser on.

Instructions for candle diffusers:

1. Pour a few tablespoons of lukewarm water into the dish.

2. Add the wintergreen and wild orange essential oils and light the candle.

Chapter 45 – Sleep Well

Ingredients:

2 drops Chamomile essential oil

2 drops Lavender essential oil

2 drops Vetiver essential oil

Instructions for ultrasonic diffusers:

1. Pour enough lukewarm water to fill the diffuser dish half the fill-line or up to the fill-line depending on how strong you want the fragrance to be.

2. Add the chamomile, lavender, vetiver essential oils and put the lid back on. Press the power button to turn the diffuser on.

Instructions for candle diffusers:

1. Pour a few tablespoons of lukewarm water into the dish.

2. Add the chamomile, lavender, vetiver essential oils and light the candle.

Conclusion

Diffusing essential oils is an easy and effective way to make use of all those incredible healing properties which these oils posses. In this book, you have read about two methods of diffusing essential oils – candle oil and ultrasonic diffusers. Moreover, the book gives you a whole variety of blends that you can try out and fill your hcme with heavenly fragrances. Hope you will find how beneficial these essential oil blends can be. Enjoy!

www.ingramcontent.com/pod-product-compliance
Lightning Source LLC
Chambersburg PA
CBHW072048280526
45788CB00006B/2226